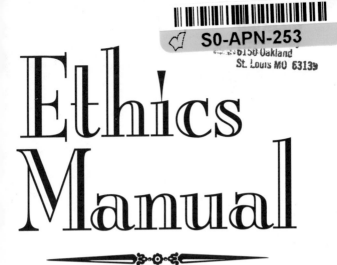

Ethics Manual

Fifth Edition

American College of Physicians

ACP Ethics and Human Rights Committee
William E. Golden, MD (Chair); Harmon H. Davis, II, MD (Vice Chair); David A. Fleming, MD; Susan E. Glennon, MD; Vincent E. Herrin, MD; Virginia L. Hood, MD, MPH; Jay A. Jacobson, MD; Stephen R. Jones, MD; Allen S. Keller, MD; Joanne Lynn, MD; Clement J. McDonald, MD; Paul S. Mueller, MD; Steven Z. Pantilat, MD; David W. Potts, MD; and Daniel P. Sulmasy, OFM, MD, PhD

Staff Authors and Editors
Lois Snyder, JD, and Cathy Leffler, JD

American College of Physicians
Philadelphia, Pennsylvania

Reprinted from *Annals of Internal Medicine* 2005;142:561-83.

ISBN: 1-930513-65-8

05 06 07 08 09 10 9 8 7 6 5 4 3 2 1

TABLE OF CONTENTS

Acknowledgments

The American College of Physicians and the ACP Ethics and Human Rights Committee are solely responsible for the contents of the Manual. Both thank former Committee members who made contributions to the development of this Manual through their reviews of drafts and work on previous editions: Troyen A. Brennan, MD; Richard J. Carroll, MD; Kenneth V. Eden, MD; Saul J. Farber, MD; Arthur W. Feinberg, MD; Steven Miles, MD; Gail J. Povar, MD; William A. Reynolds, MD; Bernard M. Rosof, MD; David L. Schiedermayer, MD; Gerald E. Thomson, MD; James A. Tulsky, MD. They also thank additional reviewers of the Manual: Dan Brock, PhD; Linda Hawes Clever, MD; Martin L. Evers, MD; Michelina Fato, MD; Robert L. Fine, MD; Charles L. Junkerman, MD; Walter J. McDonald, MD; Richard L. Neubauer, MD; Henry S. Perkins, MD; Robert L. Potter, MD; Ralph Schmeltz, MD; James R. Webster Jr., MD. Finally, they thank Emily Mok for research assistance and Laura Gregory for administrative support.

Medicine, law, and social values are not static. Re-examining the ethical tenets of medical practice and their application in new circumstances is a necessary exercise. The fifth edition of the College's Ethics Manual covers emerging issues in medical ethics and revisits old ones. It reflects on many of the ethical tensions faced by internists and their patients and attempts to shed light on how existing principles extend to emerging concerns. In addition, by reiterating ethical principles that have provided guidance in resolving past ethical problems, the Manual may help physicians avert future problems. The Manual is not a substitute for the experience and integrity of individual physicians, but it may serve as a reminder of the shared obligations and duties of the medical profession.

The secret of the care of the patient is in caring for the patient.
—Francis Weld Peabody (1)

Introduction

Some aspects of medicine are fundamental and timeless. Medical practice, however, does not stand still. Clinicians must be prepared to deal with changes and reaffirm what is fundamental. This fifth edition of the Ethics Manual examines emerging issues in medical ethics and revisits older issues that remain pertinent. Changes to the Manual since the 1998 (fourth) edition include new or expanded sections on professionalism, the physician and patient, third-party evaluations, confidentiality, complementary and alternative care, boundaries and privacy, gifts from patients, care of patients at the end of life, solid organ transplantation, physician-assisted suicide, the changing practice environment and managed care ethics, physician-industry issues, selling products out of the office, health and human rights, patient safety, prisoners as patients, strikes and joint actions, consultation and shared care, and research ethics. A case method for ethics decision making is included (see Appendix).

The Manual is intended to facilitate the process of making ethical decisions in clinical practice and medical research and to describe and explain underlying principles of decision making. Because ethics must be understood within a historical and cultural context, the second edition of the Manual included a brief overview of the cultural, philosophical, and religious underpinnings of medical ethics. In this edition, we refer the reader to that overview (2, 3) and to other sources (4–9) that more fully explore the rich heritage of medical ethics.

The Manual raises ethical issues and presents general guidelines. In applying these guidelines, physicians should consider the circumstances of the individual patient at issue and use their best judgment. Physicians have moral and legal obligations, and the two may not be concordant. Physician participation in torture is legal in some countries but is never morally defensible. Physicians must keep in mind the distinctions and potential conflicts between legal and ethical obligations when making clinical decisions and should seek counsel when they are concerned about the potential legal consequences of decisions. We refer to the law in this Manual for illustrative purposes only; these references should not be taken as a statement of the law or of the legal consequences of a physician's actions, which can vary from state to state. Physicians must develop and maintain an adequate knowledge of key components of the laws and regulations that affect their patients and practices.

Medical and professional ethics often establish positive duties (that is, what one should do) to a greater extent than the law. Current understanding of medical ethics is based on the principles from which positive duties emerge. These principles include beneficence (a duty to promote good and act in the best interest of the patient and the health of society) and nonmaleficence (the duty to do no harm to patients). Also included is respect for patient autonomy—the duty to protect and foster a patient's free, uncoerced choices (10). From the principle of respect for autonomy are derived the rules for truth-telling. The relative weight granted to these principles and the conflicts among them often account for the ethical dilemmas physicians face. Physicians who will be challenged to resolve those dilemmas must have such virtues as compassion, courage, and patience in all aspects of their practice.

In addition, considerations of justice must inform the physician's role as citizen and clinical decisions about resource allocation. The principle of distributive justice requires that we seek to equitably distribute the life-enhancing opportunities afforded by health care. How to accomplish this distribution is the focus of intense debate. More than ever, concerns about justice challenge the traditional role of physician as patient advocate.

The environment for the delivery of health care continues to change. Sites of care are shifting, with progressively more care being provided in ambulatory settings while the intensity of inpatient care continues to increase. Yet the U.S. health care system does not serve all of its citizens well, and major reform is needed. Health care financing is a serious concern, and society's values will be tested in decisions about resource allocation.

Ethical issues attract widespread public attention, and debate about them is covered regularly in the press. Through legislation, administrative action, or judicial decision, government is increasingly involved in medical ethics. Today, the convergence of various forces—scientific advances, patient and public education, the Internet, the civil rights and consumer movements, the effects of law and economics on medicine, and the heterogeneity of our society—-demands that physicians clearly articulate the ethical principles that guide their behavior, whether in clinical care, research, and teaching or as citizens. It is crucial that a responsible physician perspective be heard as societal decisions are made.

From genetic testing before conception to dilemmas at the end of life, physicians, patients, and their families are called upon to make difficult ethical decisions. The 1970s saw the development of bioethics as a field, followed by a series of reports from the U.S. President's Commission for the Study of Ethical Problems in Medicine and Biomedical and Behavioral Research. Important issues then (and now) include informed consent (11, 12), access to health care (13), genetic screening and engineering (14, 15), and forgoing life-sustaining treatment (16, 17). These and other issues—-AIDS, physician-assisted suicide, technological changes, including increasing computerization of medical records, and the physician as entrepreneur— challenge us to periodically reconsider such topics as the patient–physician relationship, decisions to limit treatment, and confidentiality.

This Manual was written for our colleagues in medicine. The College believes that the Manual provides the best approach to the challenges addressed in it. We hope that it will stimulate reasoned debate and serve as a reference for persons who seek the College's position on ethical issues. Debates about medical ethics may also stimulate critical evaluation and discussion of law and public policy on the difficult ethical issues facing patients, physicians, and society.

Professionalism

Medicine is not a trade to be learned, but a profession to be entered (1). A profession is characterized by a specialized body of knowledge that its members must teach and expand, by a code of ethics and a duty of service that put patient care above self-interest, and by the privilege of self-regulation granted by society (18). Physicians must individually and collectively fulfill the duties of the profession. While outside influences on medicine and the patient–physician relationship are many, the ethical foundations of the profession must remain in sharp focus (19).

The Physician and the Patient

The patient–physician relationship entails special obligations for the physician to serve the patient's interest because of the specialized knowledge that physicians possess and the imbalance of power caused by the medical relationship.

The physician's primary commitment must always be to the patient's welfare and best interests, whether the physician is preventing or treating illness or helping patients to cope with illness, disability, and death. The physician must respect the dignity of all persons and respect their uniqueness. The interests of the patient should always be promoted regardless of financial arrangements, the health care setting, or patient characteristics, such as decision-making capacity or social status.

At the beginning of and throughout the patient-physician relationship, the physician must work toward an understanding of the patient's health problems, concerns, goals, and expectations. After patient and physician agree on the problem and the goal of therapy, the physician presents one or more courses of action. If both parties agree, the patient may authorize the physician to initiate a course of action; the physician can then accept that responsibility. The relationship has mutual obligations. The physician must be professionally competent, act responsibly, seek consultation when necessary, and treat the patient with compassion and respect. In turn, the patient should participate responsibly in the care, including giving informed consent or refusal to care as the case might be. Effective communication is critical to a strong patient-physician relationship. Communication through means such as e-mail can supplement face-to-face encounters; however, it must be done under appropriate guidelines (20) and may not be effective for some patients.

Care and respect should guide the performance of the physical examination. The location and degree of privacy should be appropriate for the examination being performed. A chaperone should be offered to the patient or requested by the physician for physical examinations as needed. An appropriate setting and sufficient time should be allocated to encourage exploration of aspects of the patient's life pertinent to health, including habits, relationships, sexuality, vocation, religion, and spirituality.

Although the physician should be fairly compensated for services rendered, a sense of duty to the patient should take precedence over concern about compensation.

Initiating and Discontinuing the Patient-Physician Relationship

By history, tradition, and professional oath, physicians have a moral obligation to provide care for ill persons. Although this obligation is collective, each individual physician is obliged to do his or her fair share to ensure that all ill persons receive appropriate treatment (21). A physician may not discriminate against a class or category of patients.

An individual patient-physician relationship is formed on the basis of mutual agreement. In the absence of a preexisting relationship, the physician is not ethically obliged to provide care to an individual person unless no other physician is available, as is the case in some isolated communities or when emergency treatment is required. Under these circumstances, the physician is morally bound to provide care and, if necessary, to arrange for proper follow-up. Physicians may also be bound by contract to provide care to beneficiaries of health plans in which they participate.

Physicians and patients may have different concepts of the meaning and resolution of medical problems. The care of the patient and satisfaction of both parties are best served if physician and patient discuss their expectations and concerns. Although the physician must address the patient's concerns, he or she is not required to violate fundamental personal values, standards of medical care or ethical practice, or the law. When the patient's beliefs—religious, cultural, or otherwise—run counter to medical recommendations, the physician is obliged to try to understand clearly the beliefs and the viewpoints of the patient. If the physician cannot carry out the patient's wishes after seriously attempting to resolve differences, the physician should consider transferring the care of the patient.

Under exceptional circumstances, the physician may discontinue the professional relationship, provided that adequate care is available elsewhere and the patient's health is not jeopardized in the process. The physician should notify the patient in writing and obtain patient approval to transfer the medical records to another physician. Continuity of care must be assured. Abandonment is unethical and a cause of action under the law. Physician-initiated termination is a serious event, especially if the patient is acutely ill, and should be undertaken only after genuine attempts are made to understand and resolve differences. A patient is free to change physicians at any time and is entitled to the information contained in the medical records.

Third-Party Evaluations

Seeing patients on behalf of a third party, as an industry-employed physician or an independent medical examiner, raises distinct ethical issues regarding the patient-physician relationship. Within these contexts, the physician should disclose to the patient when an examination is being undertaken on behalf of a third party; ensure that the patient is aware that traditional aspects of the patient-physician relationship, including confidentiality, might not apply; obtain the examinee's consent to the examination and to the disclosure of the results to the third party; exercise appropriate independent medical judgment, free from the influence of the third party; and inform the examinee of the examination results and encourage her or him to see another physician if those results suggest the need for medical consultation (22,23).

Confidentiality

Confidentiality is a fundamental tenet of medical care. It is increasingly difficult to maintain in this era of computerized record keeping and electronic data processing, e-mail, faxing of patient information, third-party payment for medical services, and sharing of patient care among numerous health professionals and institutions. Confidentiality is a matter of respecting the privacy of patients, encouraging them to seek medical care and discuss their problems candidly, and preventing discrimination on the basis of their medical conditions. The physician should not release a patient's personal medical information (often termed a "privileged communication") without that patient's consent.

However, confidentiality, like other ethical duties, is not absolute. It may have to be overridden to protect individuals or the public or to disclose or report information when the law requires it. The physician should make every effort to discuss the issues with the patient. If breaching confidentiality is necessary, it should be done in a way that minimizes harm to the patient and that heeds applicable federal and state law.

Physicians should be aware of the increased risk for invasion of patient privacy and should help ensure confidentiality. They should be aware of state and federal legal requirements, including the Health Insurance Portability and Accountability Act of 1996 (HIPAA) Privacy Rule (24,25). Within their own institutions, physicians should advocate policies and procedures to secure the confidentiality of patient records.

To uphold professionalism and protect patient privacy, clinicians should limit discussion of patients and patient care issues to professional encounters. Discussion of patients by professional staff in public places such as elevators or cafeterias violates confidentiality and is unethical. Outside of an educational setting, discussion of patients with or near persons who are not involved in the care of those patients impairs the public's trust and confidence in the medical profession. Physicians of patients who are well known to the public should remember that they are not free to discuss or disclose information about any patient's health without the explicit consent of the patient.

In the care of the adolescent patient, family support is important. However, this support must be balanced with confidentiality and respect for the adolescent's autonomy in health care decisions and in relationships with health care providers (26). Physicians should be knowledgeable about state laws governing the right of adolescent patients to confidentiality and the adolescent's legal right to consent to treatment.

Occasionally, a physician receives information from a patient's friends or relatives and is asked to withhold the source of that information from the patient (27). The physician is not obliged to keep such secrets from the patient. The informant should be urged to address the patient directly and to encourage the patient to discuss the information with the physician. The physician should use sensitivity and judgment in deciding whether to use the information and whether to reveal its source to the patient. The physician should always act in the best interests of the patient.

The Patient and the Medical Record

Medical records should contain accurate and complete information. Ethically and legally, patients have the right to know what is in their medical records. Legally, the actual chart is the property of the physician or institution, although the information in the chart is the property of the patient. Most states have laws that guarantee the patient personal access to the medical record, as does the federal HIPAA Privacy Rule. The physician must release information to the patient or to a third party at the request of the patient. Information may not be withheld because of nonpayment of medical bills. Physicians should retain the original of the medical record and respond to a patient's request with copies or summaries as appropriate unless the original record is required. To protect confidentiality, information should be released only with the written permission of the patient or the patient's legally authorized representative, or as required under applicable law. If a physician leaves a group practice or dies, patients must be notified and records forwarded according to patient instructions.

Disclosure

To make health care decisions and work intelligently in partnership with the physician, the patient must be well informed. Effective patient-physician communication can dispel uncertainty and fear and enhance healing and patient satisfaction. Information should be disclosed whenever it is considered material to the patient's understanding of his or her situation, possible treatments, and probable outcomes. This information often includes the costs and burdens of treatment, the experience of the proposed clinician, the nature of the illness, and potential treatments.

However uncomfortable for the clinician, information that is essential to and desired by the patient must be disclosed. How and when to disclose information, and to whom, are important concerns that must be addressed with respect for patient wishes. Western tradition focuses on the rights of the individual and full and detailed disclosure. Some patients, however, may make it known that they prefer limited information, or disclosure to family members (28).

Information should be given in terms that the patient can understand. The physician should be sensitive to the patient's responses in setting the pace of communication, particularly if the illness is very serious. Disclosure and communication of health information should never be a mechanical or perfunctory process. Upsetting news and information should be presented to the patient in a way that minimizes distress (29,30). If the patient cannot comprehend his or her condition, it should be fully disclosed to an appropriate surrogate.

In addition, physicians should disclose to patients information about procedural or judgment errors made in the course of care if such information is material to the patient's well-being. Errors do not necessarily constitute improper, negligent, or unethical behavior, but failure to disclose them may.

Informed Consent

The patient's consent allows the physician to provide care. The unauthorized touching of a person is battery, even in the medical setting. Consent may be either expressed or implied. Expressed consent most often occurs in the hospital setting, where patients provide written or oral consent for a particular procedure. In many medical encounters, when the patient presents to a physician for evaluation and care, consent can be presumed. The underlying condition and treatment options are explained to the patient or authorized surrogate and treatment is rendered or refused. In medical emergencies, consent to treatment that is necessary to maintain life or restore health is usually implied unless it is known that the patient would refuse the intervention.

The doctrine of informed consent goes beyond the question of whether consent was given for a treatment or intervention. Rather, it focuses on the content and process of consent. The physician is required to provide enough information to allow a patient to make an informed judgment about how to proceed. The physician's presentation should be understandable to the patient and should include the physician's recommendation. The patient's or surrogate's concurrence must be free and uncoerced.

The principle and practice of informed consent rely on patients to ask questions when they are uncertain about the information they receive; to think carefully about their choices; and to be forthright with their physicians about their values, concerns, and reservations about a particular recommendation. Once patients and physicians decide on a course of action, patients should make every reasonable effort to carry out the aspects of care that are in their control or to inform their physicians promptly if it is not possible to do so.

The physician is obligated to ensure that the patient or the surrogate is adequately informed about the nature of the patient's medical condition and the objectives of, alternatives to, possible outcomes of, and risks involved with a proposed treatment.

All adult patients are considered competent to make decisions about medical care unless a court declares them incompetent. In clinical practice, however, physicians and family members usually make decisions without a formal competency hearing in the court for patients who lack decision-making capacity (that is, the ability to receive and express information and to make a choice consonant with that information and one's values). This clinical approach can be ethically justified if the physician has carefully determined that the patient is incapable of understanding the nature of the proposed treatment; the alternatives to it; and the risks, benefits, and consequences of it. Assessing a patient's understanding can be difficult. Decision-making capacity should be evaluated for a particular decision at a particular point in time. The capacity to express a particular goal or wish can exist without the ability to make more complex decisions. The graver the consequences of the decision, the greater the proof of capacity the physician should require.

When a patient lacks decision-making capacity, an appropriate surrogate should make decisions with the physician. Ideally, surrogate decision makers should know the patient's preferences and act in the best interests of the patient. If the patient has designated a proxy, as through a durable power of attorney for health care, that choice should be respected. When patients have not selected surrogates, standard clinical practice is that family members serve as surrogates. Some states have health care consent statutes that specify who and in what order of priority family members or friends can serve as surrogates. Physicians should be aware of legal requirements in their states for surrogate appointment and decision making. In some cases, all parties may agree that a close friend is a more appropriate surrogate than a relative.

Surrogate preferences can conflict with the preferences and best interests of a patient. Physicians should take reasonable care to ensure that the surrogate's decisions are consistent with those preferences and best interests. When possible, these decisions should be reached in the medical setting by physicians, surrogates, and other caregivers. Physicians should emphasize to surrogates that decisions should be based on what the patient would want, not what surrogates would choose for themselves. If disagreements cannot be resolved, hospital ethics committees may be helpful. Courts should be used when doing so serves the patient, such as to establish guardianship for an unbefriended, incompetent patient; to resolve a problem when other processes fail; or to comply with state law.

Surrogate decision making is best done with evidence of the patient's wishes. Physicians should routinely encourage patients to discuss their future wishes with appropriate family and friends and to complete a living will and/or durable power of attorney for health care (31,32). (See also "Advance Care Planning" in the "Care of Patients Near the End of Life" section.)

Most adult patients can participate in, and thereby share responsibility for, their health care. Physicians cannot properly diagnose and treat conditions without full information about the patient's personal and family medical history, habits, ongoing treatments (medical and otherwise), and symptoms. The physician's obligation of confidentiality exists in part to ensure that patients can be candid without fear of loss of privacy. Physicians must strive to create an environment in which honesty can thrive and patients feel concerns and questions are elicited.

Decisions About Reproduction

The ethical duty to disclose relevant information about human reproduction to the patient may conflict with the physician's personal moral standards on abortion, sterilization, contraception, or other reproductive services. A physician who objects to these services is not obligated to recommend, perform, or prescribe them. As in any other medical situation, however, the physician has a duty to inform the patient about care options and alternatives, or refer the patient for such information, so that the patient's rights are not constrained. Physicians unable to provide such information should transfer care as long as the health of the patient is not compromised.

If a patient who is a minor requests termination of pregnancy, advice on contraception, or treatment of sexually transmitted diseases without a parent's knowledge or permission, the physician may wish to attempt to persuade the patient of the benefits of having parents involved, but should be aware that a conflict may exist between the legal duty to maintain confidentiality and the obligation toward parents or guardians. Information should not be disclosed to others without the patient's permission (33). In such cases, the physician should be guided by the minor's best interest in light of the physician's conscience and responsibilities under the law.

Genetic Testing

Presymptomatic and diagnostic testing raises issues of education, counseling, confidentiality, cost, and justice. Such testing may allow clinicians to predict diseases or detect susceptibility at a time when medicine may not have the ability to prevent or cure the conditions identified. The public and health care professionals often have a limited understanding of the distinction between prediction and susceptibility or risk. Genetic testing presents unique problems by identifying risk for disease that has special meaning for patients and clinicians, as well as for family members who may not be under the care of the clinician providing the test.

Because the number of qualified clinical geneticists and genetic counselors is small and unlikely to meet the demand generated by the exponential growth in genetic testing, clinicians will be increasingly expected to convey the meaning of genetic test results. Only physicians who have the skills necessary for pretest and post-test education and counseling should engage in genetic testing (34,35). If qualified, clinicians should discuss with patients the degree to which a particular genetic risk factor correlates with the likelihood of developing disease. If unqualified or unsure, the clinician should refer the patient for this discussion. Testing should not be undertaken until the potential consequences of learning genetic information are fully discussed with the patient. The potential impact on the patient's well-being; implications for family members; and the potential for adverse use of such information by employers, insurers, or other societal institutions should be fully explored and understood.

As more information becomes available on the genetic risk for certain diseases, physicians must be aware of the need for confidentiality concerning genetic information. Many state governments and the federal government are promulgating rules that cover access of employers and insurers to such information. Additional complex ethical problems exist, such as which family members should be informed of the results of genetic tests. Physicians should be sensitive to these ethical problems, and testing should not be undertaken until these issues are fully discussed and their consequences are well understood.

The potential for stigmatization and insurance and job discrimination require that physicians ensure the confidentiality of data. However, the presence of a genetic risk factor or genetic disease in a family member raises the possibility that other genetically related individuals are at risk. The physician should encourage the affected patient's cooperation in contacting potentially affected family members or obtain the patient's consent to contact them to encourage them to seek genetic counseling.

Medical Risk to Physician and Patient

Traditionally, the ethical imperative for physicians to provide care has overridden the risk to the treating physician, even during epidemics. In recent decades, with better control of such risks, physicians have practiced medicine in the absence of risk as a prominent concern. However, potential occupational exposures such as HIV, multidrug-resistant tuberculosis, severe acute respiratory syndrome, and viral hepatitis necessitate reaffirmation of the ethical imperative (36).

Physicians should evaluate their risk for becoming infected with pathogens, both in their personal lives and in the workplace, and implement appropriate precautions. Physicians who may have been exposed to pathogens have an ethical obligation to be tested and should do so voluntarily. Infected physicians should place themselves under the guidance of their personal physician or the review of local experts to determine in a confidential manner whether practice restrictions are appropriate on the basis of the physician's specialty, compliance with infection control precautions, and physical and mental fitness to work. Infection does not in itself justify restrictions on the practice of an otherwise competent health care worker. Health care workers are expected to comply with public health and institutional policies.

Because the diseases mentioned above may be transmitted from patient to physician and because they pose significant risks to physicians' health, some physicians may be tempted to avoid the care of infected patients. Physicians and health care organizations are obligated to provide competent and humane care to all patients, regardless of their illness. Physicians can and should expect their workplace to provide appropriate means to limit occupational exposure through rigorous application of infection control methods. The denial of appropriate care to a class of patients for any reason, including disease state, is unethical (37).

Whether infected physicians should disclose their condition depends on the likelihood of risk to the patient and relevant law or regulations in their locales. Physicians should remove themselves from care if it becomes clear that the risk associated with contact or with a procedure is significant despite appropriate preventive measures. Physicians are obligated to disclose their condition after the fact if a clinically significant exposure has taken place.

Physicians have several obligations concerning nosocomial risk for infection. They should help the public understand the low level of this risk and put it in the perspective of other medical risks while acknowledging public concern. Physicians provide medical care to health care workers, and part of this care is discussing with those workers their ethical obligations to know their risk for such diseases as HIV or viral hepatitis, to voluntarily seek testing if they are at risk, and to take reasonable steps to protect patients. The physician who provides care for a seropositive health care worker must determine that worker's fitness to work. In some cases, seropositive health care workers cannot be persuaded to comply with accepted infection control guidelines, or impaired physicians cannot be persuaded to restrict their practices. In such exceptional cases, the treating physician may need to breach confidentiality and report the situation to the appropriate authorities in order to protect patients and maintain public trust in the profession, even though such actions may have legal consequences.

Complementary and Alternative Care

Complementary and alternative medicine, as defined by the National Center for Complementary and Alternative Medicine, "is a group of diverse medical and health care systems, practices, and products that are not presently considered to be part of conventional medicine" (38). Folk healing practices are also common in many cultures (39).

Requests by patients for alternative treatment require balancing the medical standard of care with a patient's right to choose care on the basis of his or her values and preferences. Such requests warrant careful physician attention. Before advising a patient, the physician should ascertain the reason for the request. The physician should be sure that the patient understands his or her condition, standard medical treatment options, and expected outcomes. Because most patients do not affirmatively disclose their use of complementary and alternative care, physicians should ask patients about their current practices (40).

The physician should encourage the patient who is using or requesting alternative treatment to seek literature and information from reliable sources (41). The patient should be clearly informed if the option under consideration is likely to delay access to effective treatment or is known to be harmful. The physician should be aware of the potential impact of alternative treatment on the patient's care. The patient's decision to select alternative forms of treatment should not alone be cause to sever the patient-physician relationship.

Disability Certification

Some patients have chronic, overwhelming, or catastrophic illnesses. In these cases, society permits physicians to justify exemption from work and to legitimize other forms of financial support. In keeping with the role of patient advocate, a physician may need to help a patient who is medically disabled obtain the appropriate disability status. Disability evaluation forms should be completed factually, honestly, and promptly.

Physicians will often find themselves confronted with a patient whose problems may not fit standard definitions of disability but who nevertheless seems deserving of assistance (for example, the patient may have very limited resources or poor housing). Physicians should not distort medical information or misrepresent the patient's functional status in an attempt to help patients. Doing so jeopardizes the trustworthiness of the physician, as well as his or her ability to advocate for patients who truly meet disability or exemption criteria.

Care of the Physician's Family, Friends, and Employees

Physicians should avoid treating themselves, close friends, or members of their own families. Physicians should also be very cautious about assuming the care of closely associated employees. Problems may include inadequate history taking or physical examination, or incomplete counseling on sensitive issues. The physician's emotional proximity can result in a loss of objectivity, or the needs of the patient may not fall within the physician's area of expertise (42). If a physician does treat a close friend, family member, or employee out of necessity, the patient should be transferred to another physician as soon as it is practicable. Otherwise, requests for care on the part of employees, family members, or friends should be resolved by helping them obtain appropriate care. Fulfilling the role of informed and loving adviser, however, is not precluded.

Sexual Contact Between Physician and Patient

Issues of dependency, trust, and transference and inequalities of power lead to increased vulnerability on the part of the patient and require that a physician not engage in a sexual relationship with a patient. It is unethical for a physician to become sexually involved with a current patient even if the patient initiates or consents to the contact.

Even sexual involvement between physicians and former patients raises concern. The impact of the patient-physician relationship may be viewed very differently by physicians and former patients, and either party may underestimate the influence of the past professional relationship. Many former patients continue to feel dependency and transference toward their physicians long after the professional relationship has ended. The intense trust often established between physician and patient may amplify the patient's vulnerability in a subsequent sexual relationship. A sexual relationship with a former patient is unethical if the physician "uses or exploits the trust, knowledge, emotions or influence derived from the previous professional relationship" (43). Because it may be difficult for the physician to judge the impact of the previous professional relationship, the physician should consult with a colleague or other professional before becoming sexually involved with a former patient (44).

Boundaries and Privacy

The presence of a chaperone during a physical examination may contribute to patient and physician comfort because of particular cultural or gender issues. In appropriate situations, physicians should ask patients if they prefer to have a chaperone present. Discussion of confidential patient information must be kept to a minimum during chaperoned examinations.

Gifts from Patients

In deciding whether to accept a gift from a patient, the physician should consider the nature of the gift, the potential implications for the patient-physician relationship, and the patient's probable motivation and expectations. A small gift to a physician as a token of appreciation is not ethically problematic. Favored treatment as a result of acceptance of any gift is problematic and undermines professionalism. It may also interfere with objectivity in the care of the patient (45).

Care of Patients Near the End of Life

End-of-life care is an important aspect of medical practice. Individual physicians and the medical community must be committed to the compassionate and competent provision of care to dying patients and their families (46) and to effective communication with patients and families (32,47). Patients rightfully expect their physicians to care for them and provide medical assistance as they live with eventually fatal illnesses. Good symptom control; ongoing commitment to serve the patient and family; and physical, psychological, and spiritual support are the hallmarks of high-quality end-of-life care. Care of patients near the end of life, however, has a moral, psychological, and interpersonal intensity that distinguishes it from most other clinical encounters.

Patients Near the End of Life

Palliative care near the end of life entails addressing physical, psychosocial, and spiritual needs and understanding that patients may at times require palliative treatment in an acute care context (48-50). To provide palliative care, the physician must be up to date on the proper use of medications and treatments, including opioids and the legality and propriety of using high doses of opioids as necessary to relieve suffering. The physician should know how to refer patients to appropriate palliative care specialists and programs, know how to use home-based and institution-based hospice care, and be aware of the palliative care abilities of the nursing homes to which patients are referred.

Families of patients near the end of life should also be prepared for the course of illness and care options at the end of life (51). When clinicians perform cardiopulmonary resuscitation, family members should usually have the choice to be present. Cultural differences at the end of life must be respected by physicians just as in other types of care. Differences in beliefs, values, and health care practices may prove challenging to physicians, depending on their comfort and experience with cultural differences (28,39). Clinicians should also be able to assist family members and loved ones experiencing grief after the death of the patient (52).

Making Decisions Near the End of Life

Informed adults with decision-making capacity have the legal and ethical right to refuse recommended life-sustaining medical treatments (53). The patient has this right regardless of whether he or she is terminally or irreversibly ill, has dependents, or is pregnant. The patient's right is based on the philosophical concept of respect for autonomy, the common-law right of self-determination, and the patient's liberty interest under the U.S. Constitution (54).

Many patients, particularly those with terminal or irreversible illness, elect to forgo certain treatments or pursue treatments, even though these are decisions that their physicians may consider unwise. These situations demand empathy, thoughtful exploration of all possibilities, negotiation, or compromise and may require time-limited trials and additional consultations.

In the unusual circumstance that no evidence shows that a specific treatment desired by the patient will provide any benefit from any perspective, the physician need not provide such treatment. The more common and much more difficult circumstance occurs when the treatment will offer some small prospect of benefit at a great burden of suffering or financial cost, but the patient or family nevertheless desires it. If the physician and patient (or appropriate surrogate) cannot agree on how to proceed, there is no easy, automatic solution. Consultation with colleagues or with an ethics committee may be helpful. Timely transfer of care to another care provider who is willing to pursue the patient's preference may resolve the problem. Infrequently, legal recourse may be necessary.

Patients without decision-making capacity (see the section on informed consent) have the same rights concerning life-sustaining treatment decisions as mentally competent patients. Treatment should conform to what the patient would want on the basis of written or oral advance care planning. If these preferences are not known, care decisions should be based on the best evidence of what the patient would have chosen (substituted judgments) or, failing that, on the best interests of the patient. Physicians should be aware that hospital protocols and state legal requirements affecting end-of-life care vary.

Advance Care Planning

Advance care planning allows a competent person to indicate preferences for care and choose a surrogate to act on his or her behalf in the event that he or she cannot make health care decisions. It allows the patient's values and circumstances to shape the plan and allows specific arrangements to be made to ensure implementation of the plan.

Physicians should routinely raise the issue of advance planning with competent adult patients and encourage them to review their values and preferences with their surrogates and family members. This is best done before a health care crisis. These discussions let the physician know the patient's views, enable the physician to update the medical record, and allow the physician to reassure the patient that he or she is willing to discuss these sensitive issues and will respect patient choices. The patient and the physician should develop plans to make sure patient wishes are implemented. Discussions about patient preferences should be documented in the medical record. The Patient Self-Determination Act of 1990 requires hospitals, nursing homes, health maintenance organizations, and hospices that participate in Medicare and Medicaid programs to ask if the patient has an advance directive, to provide information about advance directives, and to incorporate advance directives into the medical record.

Advance planning takes place in conversations with the physician (with documentation in the medical record) or through written advance directives, such as a living will or durable power of attorney for health care (55). The latter enables a patient to appoint a surrogate who will make decisions if the patient becomes unable to do so. The surrogate is obligated to act in accordance with the patient's previously expressed preferences or best interests.

Living wills enable persons to describe the kind of treatment they would like to receive in the event that they lose decision-making capacity. Uncertainty about a future clinical course complicates the interpretation of living wills and emphasizes the need for physicians and patients to discuss patient preferences before a crisis arises. Talking about future medical care is an effective method of planning. Some state laws limit the application of advance directives to terminal illness or deem the advance directives not applicable if, for example, the patient is pregnant. Many states have documents that combine the living will and the durable power of attorney for health care into one document. Some specify requirements for witnessing the document.

Advance directives should be readily accessible to health care professionals regardless of the site of care. In addition, some states have statewide systems for documenting physician orders on end-of-life care, such as Oregon's Physicians Orders for Life-Sustaining Treatment (POLST) form (56). When there is no advance directive and the patient's values and preferences are unknown or unclear, decisions should be based on the patient's best interests whenever possible, as interpreted by a guardian or, if available, by a person with loving knowledge of the patient. When making the decision to forgo treatment, many people give the most weight to reversibility of disease or dependence on life support, loss of capacity for social interaction, or nearness to death. Family members and health care workers should avoid projecting their own values or views about quality of life onto the incapacitated patient. Quality of life should be assessed according to the patient's perspective (57,58).

Withdrawing or Withholding Treatment

Withdrawing and withholding treatment are equally justifiable, ethically and legally. Treatments should not be withheld because of the mistaken fear that if they are started, they cannot be withdrawn. This practice would deny patients potentially beneficial therapies. Instead, a time-limited trial of therapy could be used to clarify the patient's prognosis. At the end of the trial, a conference to review and revise the treatment plan should be held. Some health care workers or family members may be reluctant to withdraw treatments even when they believe that the patient would not have wanted them continued. The physician should try to prevent or resolve these situations by addressing with families their feelings of guilt, fear, and concern that the patient may suffer as life support is withdrawn.

Do-Not-Resuscitate Orders

Intervention in the case of a cardiopulmonary arrest is inappropriate for some patients, particularly those with terminal irreversible illness whose death is expected and imminent. Because the onset of cardiopulmonary arrest does not permit deliberative decision making, decisions about resuscitation must be made in advance. Physicians should especially encourage patients who face serious illness or who are of advanced age, or their surrogates, to discuss resuscitation.

Although a do-not-resuscitate order applies only to cardiopulmonary resuscitation, discussions about this issue often reflect a revision of the larger goals and means of the care plan. The entire health care team must be carefully apprised of the nature of these changes. Do-not-resuscitate orders or requests for no cardiopulmonary resuscitation should specify care strategies and must be written in the medical record along with notes and orders that describe all other changes in the treatment goals or plans. It is essential that patients or surrogates understand that a do-not-resuscitate order does not mean that the patient will be ineligible for other life-prolonging measures, both therapeutic and palliative. However, the appropriateness of a do-not-resuscitate order during and immediately after a procedure needs to be individually negotiated. Because it is deceptive, physicians or nurses should not perform half-hearted resuscitation efforts ("slow codes") (59).

Sometimes a patient or surrogate insists on a resuscitation effort, even when informed that it will almost certainly fail. A family's religious or other beliefs or need for closure under such circumstances deserve careful attention. Although the physician need not provide an effort at resuscitation that cannot conceivably restore circulation and breathing, the physician should help the family to understand and accept this position. A more controversial issue is whether physicians may unilaterally write a do-not-resuscitate order when the patient may survive for a very brief time in the hospital. Some institutions, with forewarning to patients and families, allow physicians to write orders against resuscitation over the patient's or family's objections. Empathy and thoughtful exploration of options for care with patients or surrogate decision makers should make such impasses rare. Full discussion about the issue should include the indications for and outcomes of cardiopulmonary resuscitation, the physical impact on the patient, implications for caregivers, the do-not-resuscitate order, the legal aspects of such orders, and the physician's role as patient advocate. A physician who writes a unilateral do-not-resuscitate order must inform the patient or surrogate.

Any decision about advance care planning, including a decision to forgo attempts at resuscitation, should apply in every care setting for that patient. Decisions made in one setting should consider future situations and the appropriateness of applying that decision in that setting. In general, a decision to forgo attempts at resuscitation should apply in every setting—hospital, home, and nursing home. Many states and localities have systematic requirements for out-of-hospital implementation of do-not-resuscitate orders (60), and physicians should know how to effectuate the order and try to protect the patient from inappropriate resuscitation efforts. Physicians should also be attentive to ensuring that orders against trying resuscitation transfer with the patient and that subsequent care teams understand and support the decision.

Determination of Death

The irreversible cessation of all functions of the entire brain is an accepted legal standard for determining death when the use of life support precludes reliance on traditional cardiopulmonary criteria. After a patient has been declared dead by brain-death criteria, medical support should ordinarily be discontinued. In some circumstances, such as the need to preserve organs for transplantation, to counsel or accommodate family beliefs or needs, or to sustain a viable fetus, physicians may temporarily support bodily functions after death has been determined.

Solid Organ Transplantation

There is an increasingly unmet need for organs and tissues. Physicians should be involved in community efforts to make potential donors aware of their option to make a gift that would enhance life, health, or sight by organ or tissue donation. Ideally, physicians will discuss the option of organ donation with patients when discussing advance care planning as part of a routine office visit, before the need arises (61). All potential donors should communicate their preference to their families as well as have it listed on such documents as driver's licenses or organ donor cards.

While a prima facie good, organ donation requires consideration of several ethical cautions. One set of issues concerns the need to avoid even the appearance of conflict between the care of a potential donor and the needs of a potential recipient (62). The care of the potential donor must be kept separate from the care of a recipient. The potential donor's physician should not be responsible for the care of the recipient or be involved in retrieving the organs or tissue. However, the potential donor's physician may alert an organ-tissue procurement team of the existence of a potential donor. Once brain death has occurred and organ donation is authorized, the donor's physician should know how to maintain the viability of organs and tissues in coordination with the procurement team. Before declaration of brain death, treatments proposed to maintain the function of transplantable organs may be used only if they are not expected to harm the potential donor.

Another issue concerns who should make the organ request. Under federal regulations, all families must be presented with the option of organ donation when the death of the patient is imminent. To avoid conflicts of interest, however, those who will perform the transplant or are caring for the potential recipient should not be involved in the request. Physicians caring for the potential donor should ensure that families are treated with sensitivity and compassion. Previously expressed preferences about donation by dying or brain-dead patients should be sought. However, only an organ procurement representative who has completed training by an organ procurement organization may initiate the actual request. This can include physicians, if they have received specific training (63).

A third set of issues involves the use of financial incentives to encourage organ donation. While increasing the supply of organs is a noble goal, the use of direct financial incentives raises ethical questions, including treatment of humans as commodities, and the potential for exploitation of families of limited means. Even the appearance of exploitation may ultimately be counter-productive to the goal of increasing the pool of organs. Retrospective, indirect compensation for expenses is less likely to raise such concerns.

A new set of issues has been raised by the advent of so-called non–heart-beating cadaveric organ donation. This approach allows patients who do not meet the criteria for brain death, but whose loved ones are considering the discontinuation of life support, to be considered potential organ donors. Life support may be discontinued under controlled conditions. Once the patient has met traditional cardiopulmonary criteria for death and after a suitable period of time that allows clinical certitude of death but does not unduly compromise the chances of successful transplantation, the organs can be harvested. As in organ donation from brain-dead individuals, the care of the potential donor and the request from the family must be separated from the care of the potential recipient. The decision to discontinue life support must be kept separate from the decision to donate, and the actual request can be made only by an organ procurement representative. Because these potential donors may not always die after the discontinuation of life support, it is unethical, before the declaration of death, to use a treatment aimed at preserving organs for donation if it is likely to cause symptoms or to compromise the chance of survival.

Irreversible Loss of Consciousness

Persons who are in a persistent vegetative state are unconscious (64-66) but not brain dead. They lack awareness of their surroundings and the ability to respond purposefully to them. Because a persistent vegetative state is not itself progressive, the prognosis for these patients varies with cause. Some physicians and medical societies believe that there are no medical indications for life-prolonging treatment or access to intensive care or respirators when patients are confirmed to be in a persistent vegetative state (67). They conclude that these patients cannot experience any benefits or suffer any discomfort and that all interventions should therefore be withdrawn. However, many patients or families value life in and of itself regardless of neurologic state. For these reasons, goals of care as decided by a patient in advance or by an appropriate surrogate should guide decisions about life-prolonging treatment for the patient in a persistent vegetative state in the same manner as for other patients without decision-making capacity.

Artificial Nutrition and Hydration

Artificial administration of nutrition and fluids is a medical intervention subject to the same principles of decision making as other treatments. Some states require high levels of proof before previous statements or advance directives can be accepted as firm evidence that a patient would not want these treatments, especially for patients who are not terminally ill, are not permanently unconscious, or have advanced dementia. For this reason, physicians should counsel patients to establish advance care directives and complete these parts of living wills especially carefully. Despite research findings to the contrary, there remain understandable concerns that discontinuing use of feeding tubes will cause suffering from hunger or thirst. Physicians should carefully address this issue with families and caregivers.

Physician-Assisted Suicide and Euthanasia

The debate over physician-assisted suicide is very important to physicians and patients. Both groups favor easing the dying process, providing adequate pain control, and avoiding unwanted treatments and protracted suffering. Patients and physicians may find it difficult at times to distinguish between the need for assistance in the dying process and the practice of assisting suicide.

Physician-assisted suicide occurs when a physician provides a medical means for death, usually a prescription for a lethal amount of medication that the patient takes on his or her own. In euthanasia, the physician directly and intentionally administers a substance to cause death. Physicians and patients should distinguish between a decision by a patient or authorized surrogate to refuse life-sustaining treatment or an inadvertent death during an attempt to relieve suffering, from physician-assisted suicide and euthanasia. Laws concerning or moral objections to physician-assisted suicide and euthanasia should not deter physicians from honoring a decision to withhold or withdraw medical interventions in appropriate situations. Fears that unwanted life-sustaining treatment will be imposed continue to motivate some patients to request assisted suicide or euthanasia.

In the clinical setting, all of these acts must be framed within the larger context of good end-of-life care. Many patients who request assisted suicide are depressed, have uncontrolled pain, or have potentially reversible suffering or fears (68). In the setting of providing comfort to a dying person, most physicians and patients should be able to address these issues. For example, with regard to pain control, the physician may appropriately increase medication to relieve pain, even if this action inadvertently shortens life (the "double effect") (69,70).

The College does not support legalization of physician-assisted suicide (71). After much consideration, the College concluded that making physician-assisted suicide legal raised serious ethical, clinical, and social concerns and that the practice might undermine patient trust and distract from reform in end of life care. The College was also concerned with the risks that legalization posed to vulnerable populations, including poor persons, patients with dementia, disabled persons, those from minority groups that have experienced discrimination, those confronting costly chronic illnesses, or very young children. One state, Oregon, has legalized the practice of physician-assisted suicide, and its experience is being reviewed (72,73). Other states might legalize this practice, but the major emphasis of the College and its members, including those who might lawfully participate in the practice, must focus on ensuring that all persons facing serious illness can count on good care through to the end of life, with prevention or relief of suffering, commitment to human dignity, and support for the burdens borne by family and friends. Physicians and patients must continue to search together for answers to the problems posed by the difficulties of living with serious illness before death, without violating the physician's personal and professional values, and without abandoning the patient to struggle alone.

The Ethics of Practice

The Changing Practice Environment

Many individual persons, groups, and institutions play a role in and are affected by medical decision making. In an environment characterized by increasing demand, increasing regulation and decreasing professional autonomy, mounting health care inflation, and significantly constrained resources, tension and conflict are inevitable among patients, clinicians, insurers, purchasers, government, health care institutions, and health care industries. However, all these parties have an obligation to interact honestly, openly, and fairly (74). And while this section of the Manual focuses specifically on the obligations of physicians in this changing context, it is essential to note that all of these parties bear responsibility for recognizing and supporting the intimacy and importance of relationships with patients and the ethical obligations of clinicians to patients. Further, concern about the impact of the changing practice environment on physicians and insured patients should not distract physicians or society from attending to the unmet needs of persons who lack insurance. Attention to these larger questions of quality and access will require a public dialogue in which all these parties should participate. Resource allocation decisions should always be made through an open and participatory process.

Physicians have an obligation to promote their patients' welfare in this increasingly complex health care system. This entails forthrightly helping patients to understand clinical recommendations and to make informed choices among all appropriate care options. It includes management of the conflicts of interest and multiple commitments that arise in any practice environment, especially in an era of cost concerns. It also includes stewardship of finite health care resources so that as many health care needs as possible can be met, whether in the physician's office, the hospital, or the long-term care facility or at home.

The patient-physician relationship and the principles that govern it should be central to the delivery of care. These principles include beneficence, honesty, confidentiality, privacy, and advocacy when patients' interests may be endangered by arbitrary, unjust, or inadequately individualized institutional procedures. Health care, however, does take place in a broader context beyond the patient-physician relationship. A patient's preferences or interests may conflict with the interests or values of the physician, an institution, a payer, other members of a managed care plan who have equal claim to the same health care resources, or society.

The physician's first and primary duty is to the patient. Physicians must base their counsel on the interests of the individual patient, regardless of the insurance or medical care delivery setting. Whether financial incentives in the fee-for-service system prompt physicians to do more rather than less or managed care arrangements encourage them to do less rather than more, physicians must not allow such considerations to affect their clinical judgment or patient counseling on treatment options, including referrals (75). The physician's professional role is to make recommendations on the basis of their medical merit and to pursue options that comport with the patient's unique background and preferences (76).

Physicians have a responsibility to practice effective and efficient health care and to use health care resources responsibly. Parsimonious care that utilizes the most efficient means to effectively diagnose a condition and treat a patient respects the need to use resources wisely and to help ensure that resources are equitably available. In making recommendations to patients, designing practice guidelines and formularies, and making decisions on medical benefits review boards, physicians' considered judgments should reflect the best clinical literature, including data on the cost-effectiveness of different clinical approaches. When patients ask, they should be informed of the rationale that underlies the physician's recommendation.

Health plans are not obliged to underwrite approaches that patients may value but that are not justifiable on clinical or theoretical scientific grounds or that are relatively cost-ineffective compared with other therapies for the same condition or other therapies offered by the health plan for other conditions. However, the plan must have in place a fair appeals procedure. In instances of disagreement between patient and physician for any reason, the physician is obligated to explain the basis for the disagreement, to educate the patient, and to meet the patient's needs for comfort and reassurance.

The physician's duty further requires serving as the patient's agent within the health care arena. In the managed care context, for example, advocacy can operate at many levels. At the individual-patient level, the physician advocate must pursue the necessary avenues to obtain treatment that is essential to the patient's care, regardless of the barriers that may discourage the physician from doing so. Moreover, physicians should advocate just as vigorously for the needs of their most vulnerable and disadvantaged patients as they do for their most articulate patients (74).

Patients may not understand or may fear conflicts of interest for physicians and the multiple commitments that can arise from cost-containment pressure under managed care. Physicians should disclose potential conflicts of interest to their patients. But health care plans have duties to foster an ethical practice environment, and should not ask physicians to participate in any arrangements that jeopardize professional and ethical standards. They should hold physicians accountable for the quality of care and not simply for economic performance. Physicians should enter into agreements with insurers or other organizations only if they can ensure that these agreements do not violate professional and ethical standards. Managed care plans should not restrict the information or counsel that physicians may give patients.

Although the physician must provide information to the patient about all appropriate care and referral options, the health plan must disclose all relevant information about benefits, including any restrictions, and about financial incentives that might negatively affect patient access to care (77).

When patients enroll in insurance plans, they receive a great deal of information on rules governing benefits and reimbursement. Meaningful disclosure requires explanations that are clear and easily understood. Insured patients and their families bear a responsibility for having a basic understanding of the rules of their insurance (74). Physicians cannot and should not be expected to advise patients on the particulars of individual insurance contracts and arrangements. Patients should, however, expect their physicians to honor the rules of the insurer unless doing so would endanger the patient's health. Physicians should not collaborate with a patient or engage in efforts to defraud the insurer.

Financial Arrangements

Financial relationships between patients and physicians vary from fee-for-service to government contractual arrangements and prepaid insurance. Financial arrangements and expectations should be clearly established. Fees for physician services should accurately reflect the services provided. Physicians should be aware that a beneficent intention to forgive copayments for patients who are financially stressed may nonetheless be fraud under current law.

When physicians elect to offer professional courtesy to a colleague, physicians and patients should function without feelings of constraint on time or resources and without shortcut approaches. Colleague-patients who initiate questions in informal settings put the treating physician in a less-than-ideal position to provide optimal care. Both parties should avoid this inappropriate practice.

As professionals dedicated to serving the sick, all physicians should do their fair share to provide services to uninsured and underinsured persons. Physicians who participate in retainer fee practices ("boutique" or "concierge" medicine) should be aware that by thus limiting their patient populations, they risk compromising their professional obligation to care for the poor and the credibility of medicine's commitment to serving all classes of patients who are in need of medical care (78).

Financial Conflicts of Interest

The physician must seek to ensure that the medically appropriate level of care takes primacy over financial considerations imposed by the physician's own practice, investments, or financial arrangements. Even the appearance of impropriety undermines trust in the profession.

Potential influences on clinical judgment cover a wide range and include financial incentives inherent in the practice environment (such as incentives to overutilize in the fee-for-service setting or underutilize in the managed care setting) (79,80), drug industry gifts, and business arrangements involving referrals. Physicians must be conscious of all potential influences, and their actions should be guided by patient best interests and appropriate utilization, not by other factors.

Physicians who have potential financial conflicts of interest, whether as researchers, speakers, consultants, investors, partners, employers, or otherwise, must not in any way compromise their objective clinical judgment or the best interests of patients or research subjects (81). Physicians must disclose their financial interests in any medical facilities or office-based research to which they refer or recruit patients. When speaking, teaching, and authoring, physicians with ties to a particular company should disclose their interests in writing. Most journal editors require that authors and peer reviewers disclose any potential conflicts of interest. Editors themselves should be free from conflicts of interest.

Physicians should not refer patients to an outside facility in which they have invested and at which they do not directly provide care (82). Physicians may, however, invest in or own health care facilities when capital funding and necessary services that would otherwise not be made available are provided. In such situations, in addition to disclosing these interests to patients, physicians must establish safeguards against abuse, impropriety, or the appearance of impropriety.

A fee paid to one physician by another for the referral of a patient, historically known as fee-splitting, is unethical. It is also unethical for a physician to receive a commission or a kickback from anyone, including a company that manufactures or sells medical instruments or medications that are used in the care of the physician's patients.

The sale of products from the physician's office may be considered by some patients as a form of self-referral and may negatively affect the trust necessary to sustain the patient-physician relationship. Most products should not be sold in the office, and the College has taken a position that asks physicians to consider seriously the moral issues involved in a decision to do so (83). Physicians should not sell products out of the office unless the products are specifically relevant to the patient's care, offer a clear benefit based on adequate clinical evidence and research, and meet an urgent need of the patient. If geographic or time constraints make it difficult or impracticable for patients to obtain a medically relevant and urgently needed product otherwise, selling a product in the office would be ethically acceptable. For example, a splint or crutches would be acceptable products, but vitamin supplements and cosmetic items are neither emergent treatments nor unlikely to be available elsewhere, and so the sale of such products is ethically suspect. Physicians should make full disclosure about their financial interests in selling acceptable products and inform patients about alternatives for purchasing the product. Charges for products sold through the office should be limited to the reasonable costs incurred in making them available. The selling of products intended to be free samples is unethical.

Physicians may invest in publicly traded securities. However, care must be taken to avoid investment decisions that may create a conflict of interest or the perception of a conflict of interest. The acceptance of individual gifts, hospitality, trips, and subsidies of all types from the health care industry by an individual physician is strongly discouraged. The acceptance of even small gifts has been documented to affect clinical judgment and heightens the perception (as well as the reality) of a conflict of interest (84). In addition to applying the Royal College of Physicians' standard and asking, "Would I be willing to have this arrangement generally known?" (85), physicians should also ask, "What would the public or my patients think of this arrangement?"; "What is the purpose of the industry offer?"; "What would my colleagues think about this arrangement?"; and "What would I think if my own physician accepted this offer?" (81).

Physicians must critically evaluate all medical information, including that provided by detail persons, advertisements, or industry-sponsored educational programs. While providers of public and private graduate and continuing medical education may accept industry support for educational programs, they should develop and enforce strict policies maintaining complete control of program planning, content, and delivery. They should be aware of, and vigilant against, potential bias and conflicts of interest (86).

If medical professional societies accept industry support or other external funding, they also "should be aware of potential bias and conflicts of interest and should develop and enforce explicit policies that preserve the independent judgment and professionalism of their members and maintain the ethical standards and credibility of the society" (86).

Advertising

Advertising by physicians or health care institutions is unethical when it contains statements that are unsubstantiated, false, deceptive, or misleading, including statements that mislead by omitting necessary information.

The Physician and Society

Society has conferred professional prerogatives on physicians with the expectation that they will use their position for the benefit of patients. In turn, physicians are responsible and accountable to society for their professional actions. Society grants each physician the rights, privileges, and duties pertinent to the patient-physician relationship and has the right to require that physicians be competent and knowledgeable and that they practice with consideration for the patient as a person.

Obligations of the Physician to Society

Physicians have obligations to society that in many ways parallel their obligations to individual patients. Physicians' conduct as professionals and as individuals should merit the respect of the community.

All physicians must fulfill the profession's collective responsibility to advocate the health and well-being of the public. Physicians should protect public health by reporting disease, injury, domestic violence, abuse, or neglect to the responsible authority as required by law.

Physicians should support community health education and initiatives that provide the general public with accurate information about health care and should contribute to keeping the public properly informed by commenting on medical subjects in their areas of expertise. Physicians should provide the news media with accurate information, recognizing this as an obligation to society and an extension of medical practice. However, patient confidentiality must be respected.

Physicians should help policymakers recognize and address the social and environmental causes of disease, including human rights concerns, poverty, and violence. Physicians should work toward ensuring access to health care for all persons; act to eliminate discrimination in health care; and help correct deficiencies in the availability, accessibility, and quality of health services, including mental health services, in the community. The denial of appropriate care to a class of patients for any reason is unethical. Importantly, disparities in care as a result of personal characteristics such as race have recently received increased attention and need to be addressed (87). Physicians should also explore how their own attitudes, knowledge, and beliefs may influence their ability to fulfill these obligations.

Health and human rights are interrelated. When human rights are promoted, health is promoted. Violation of human rights has harmful consequences for the individual and the community. Physicians have an important role to play in promoting health and human rights, and addressing social inequities. This includes caring for vulnerable populations, such as the uninsured and victims of violence or human rights abuses. Physicians have an opportunity and duty to advocate for the needs of individual patients as well as society.

Physicians should advocate for and participate in patient safety initiatives, including error, sentinel event, and "near-miss" reporting. Human errors in health care are not uncommon (88), and many result from systems problems. Physicians should initiate process improvement and work with their institutions and in all aspects of their practices in an ongoing effort to reduce errors and improve care.

Resource Allocation

Medical care is delivered within social and institutional systems that must take overall resources into account. Increasingly, decisions about resource allocations challenge the physician's primary role as patient advocate. This advocacy role has always had limits. For example, a physician should not lie to third-party payers for a patient in order to ensure coverage or maximize reimbursement. Moreover, a physician is not obligated to provide all treatments and diagnostics without considering their effectiveness (89) (see "The Changing Practice Environment" section). The just allocation of resources and changing reimbursement methods present the physician with ethical problems that cannot be ignored. Two principles are agreed upon:

1. As a physician performs his or her primary role as a patient's trusted advocate, he or she has a responsibility to use all health-related resources in a technically appropriate and efficient manner. He or she should plan work-ups carefully and avoid unnecessary testing, medications, surgery, and consultations.

2. Resource allocation decisions are most appropriately made at the policy level rather than entirely in the context of an individual patient-physician encounter. Ethical allocation policy is best achieved when all affected parties discuss what resources exist, to what extent they are limited, what costs attach to various benefits, and how to equitably balance all these factors.

Physicians, patient advocates, insurers, and pay-ors should participate together in decisions at the policy level; should emphasize the value of health to society; should promote justice in the health care system; and should base allocations on medical need, efficacy, cost-effectiveness, and proper distribution of benefits and burdens in society.

Relation of the Physician to Government

Physicians must not be a party to and must speak out against torture or other abuses of human rights. Participation by physicians in the execution of prisoners except to certify death is unethical. Under no circum-stances is it ethical for a physician to be used as an instrument of government to weaken the physical or mental resistance of a human being, nor should a physician participate in or tolerate cruel or unusual punishment or disciplinary activities beyond those permitted by the United Nations Standard Minimum Rules for the Treatment of Prisoners (90).

Limited access to health care is one of the most sig-nificant characteristics of correctional systems in the United States (91). Physicians who treat prisoners as patients face special challenges in balancing the best interests of the patient with those of the correctional system. Despite these limitations, physicians should advocate for timely treatment and make independent medical judgments about what constitutes appropriate care for individual inmates.

Ethics Committees and Consultants

Ethics committees and consultants contribute to achieving patient care goals by facilitating resolution of conflicts in a respectful atmosphere through a fair and inclusive decision-making process, helping institu-tions to shape policies and practices that conform with the highest ethical standards, and assisting individual persons with handling current and future ethical prob-lems by providing education in health care ethics (92).

Accrediting organizations now require most health care facilities to provide ethics consultation at the request of patients, nurses, physicians, or others (93). Physicians should be aware that this resource is available. Consultation should be guided by standards such as those developed by the American Society for Bioethics and Humanities (94). Ethics committees should be multidisciplinary and broadly representative to assure the perspectives necessary to address the complex problems with which they are confronted.

Medicine and the Law

Physicians should remember that the presence of illness does not diminish the right or expectation to be treated equally. Stated another way, illness does not in and of itself change a patient's legal rights or permit a physician to ignore those legal rights.

The law is society's mechanism for establishing boundaries for conduct. Society has a right to expect that those boundaries will not be disregarded. In instances of conflict, the physician must decide whether to violate the law for the sake of what he or she considers the dictates of medical ethics. Such a violation may jeopardize the physician's legal position or the legal rights of the patient. It should be remembered that ethical concepts are not always fully reflected in or adopted by the law. Violation of the law for purposes of complying with one's ethical standards may have significant consequences for the physician and should be undertaken only after thorough consideration and, generally, after obtaining legal counsel.

Expert Witnesses

Physicians have specialized knowledge and expertise that may be needed in judicial or administrative processes. Often, expert testimony is necessary for a court or administrative agency to understand the patient's condition, treatment, and prognosis. Physicians may be reluctant to become involved in legal proceedings because the process is unfamiliar and time-consuming. Their absence may mean, however, that legal decisions are made without the benefit of all medical facts or opinions. Without the participation of physicians, the mechanisms used to resolve many disputes may be ineffective and patients may suffer.

Although physicians cannot be compelled to participate as expert witnesses, the profession as a whole has the ethical duty to assist patients and society in resolving disputes (95). In this role, physicians must have the appropriate expertise in the subject matter of the case and honestly and objectively interpret and represent the medical facts. Physicians should accept only noncontingent compensation for the reasonable time and expenses incurred as expert witnesses.

Strikes and Other Joint Actions by Physicians

Changes in the practice environment sometimes adversely affect the ability of physicians to provide patients with high-quality care and can challenge the physician's autonomy to exercise independent clinical judgment and even the ability to sustain a practice. However, physician efforts to advocate for system change should not include participation in joint actions that adversely affect access to health care or that result in anticompetitive behavior (96). Physicians should not engage in strikes, work stoppages, slowdowns, boycotts, or other organized actions that are designed, implicitly or explicitly, to limit or deny services to patients that would otherwise be available. In general, physicians should individually and collectively find advocacy alternatives, such as lobbying lawmakers and working to educate the public, patient groups, and policymakers about their concerns. Protests and marches that constitute protected free speech and political activity can be a legitimate means to seek redress, provided that they do not involve joint decisions to engage in actions that may harm patients.

The Physician's Relationship to Other Physicians

Physicians share their commitment to care for ill persons with a broad team of health professionals. The team's ability to care effectively for the patient depends on the ability of individual persons to treat each other with integrity, honesty, and respect in daily professional interactions regardless of race, religion, ethnicity, nationality, sex, sexual orientation, age, or disability. Particular attention is warranted with regard to certain types of relationships and power imbalances that could be abusive or lead to harassment, such as those between attending physician and resident, resident and medical student, or physician and nurse (97).

Attending Physicians and Physicians-in-Training

The very title *doctor,* from the Latin *docere,* "to teach," means that physicians have a responsibility to share knowledge and information with colleagues and patients. This sharing includes teaching clinical skills and reporting results of scientific research to colleagues, medical students, resident physicians, and other health care providers.

The physician has a responsibility to teach the science, art, and ethics of medicine to medical students, resident physicians, and others and to supervise physicians in training. Attending physicians must treat trainees and colleagues with respect, empathy, and compassion. In the teaching environment, graduated authority for patient management can be delegated to residents, with adequate supervision. All trainees should inform patients of their training status and role in the medical team. Attending physicians, chiefs of service, or consultants should encourage residents to acknowledge their limitations and ask for help or supervision when concerns arise about patient care or the ability of others to perform their duties. The training environment should also encourage trainees to raise ethical issues they may encounter (98).

It is unethical to delegate authority for patient care to anyone, including another physician, who is not appropriately qualified and experienced. On a teaching service, the ultimate responsibility for patient welfare and quality of care remains with the patient's attending physician of record.

Prior permission from the patient's authorized representative to perform training procedures on newly deceased patient should be obtained in light of any known preferences of the patient regarding the handling of her or his body or the performance of such procedures.

Consultation and Shared Care

In almost all circumstances, patients should be encouraged to initially seek care from their principal physician. Physicians should in turn obtain competent consultation whenever they and their patients feel the need for assistance with care (99). The purpose, nature, and expectations of the consultation should be clear to all.

The consultant should respect the relationship between the patient and the principal physician, should promptly and effectively communicate recommendations to the principal physicians, and should obtain concurrence of the principal physician for major procedures or additional consultants. The consultant should also share his/her findings, diagnostic assessment, and recommendations with the patient. The care of the patient and the proper records should be transferred back to the principal physician when the consultation is completed, unless another arrangement is agreed upon.

Consultants who need temporary charge of the patient's care should obtain the principal physician's cooperation and assent. The physician who does not agree with the consultant's recommendations is free to call in another consultant. The interests of the patient should remain paramount in this process.

A complex clinical situation may call for multiple consultations. To assure a coordinated effort that is in the best interest of the patient, the principal physician should remain in charge of overall care, communicating with the patient and coordinating care on the basis of information derived from the consultations. Unless authority has been formally transferred elsewhere, the responsibility for the patient's care lies with the principal physician.

When the patient is in the care of a hospitalist, good communication is key. The principal physician should supply the hospitalist with adequate information about current and past clinical history to allow for appropriate decision making. The hospitalist should keep the principal physician informed of the patient's clinical course and supply that physician with a timely and complete description of care. Changes in chronic medications and plans for follow-up care should be discussed and agreed to by the principal physician before discharge.

The Impaired Physician

Physicians who are impaired for any reason must refrain from assuming patient responsibilities that they may not be able to discharge safely and effectively. Whenever there is doubt, they should seek assistance in caring for their patients.

Impairment may result from use of habit-forming agents (alcohol or other substances) or from psychiatric, physiologic, or behavioral disorders. Impairment may also be caused by diseases that affect the cognitive or motor skills necessary to provide adequate care. The presence of these disorders or the fact that a physician is being treated for them does not necessarily imply impairment.

Every physician is responsible for protecting patients from an impaired physician and for assisting an impaired colleague. Fear of mistake, embarrassment, or possible litigation should not deter or delay identification of an impaired colleague (100). The identifying physician may find it helpful to discuss the issue with the departmental chair, or a senior member of the staff or the community.

Although the legal responsibility to do so varies among states, there is a clear ethical responsibility to report a physician who seems to be impaired to an appropriate authority (such as a chief of service, chief of staff, institutional or medical society assistance program, or state medical board). Physicians should assist their impaired colleagues in identifying appropriate sources of help. While undergoing therapy, the impaired physician is entitled to full confidentiality as in any other patient-physician relationship. To protect patients of the impaired physician, someone other than the physician of the impaired physician must monitor the impaired physician's fitness to work. Serious conflicts may occur if the treating physician tries to fill both roles (101).

Peer Review

All physicians have a duty to participate in peer review. Fears of retaliation, ostracism by colleagues, loss of referrals, or inconvenience are not adequate reasons for refusing to participate in peer review. Society looks to physicians to establish and enforce professional standards of practice, and this obligation can be met only when all physicians participate in the process. Federal law and most states provide legal protection for physicians who participate in peer review in good faith.

It is unethical for a physician to disparage the professional competence, knowledge, qualifications, or services of another physician to a patient or a third party or to state or imply that a patient has been poorly managed or mistreated by a colleague without substantial evidence. However, professionalism entails membership in a self-correcting, moral community. A physician therefore has a duty to patients, the public, and the profession to report to the appropriate authority any well-formed suspicions of fraud, professional misconduct, incompetence, or abandonment of patients by another physician. Professional peer review is critical in assuring fair assessment of physician performance for the benefit of patients. The trust that patients and the public invest in physicians requires disclosure to the appropriate authorities and to patients at risk for immediate harm.

In the absence of substantial evidence of professional misconduct, negligence, or incompetence, it is unethical to use the peer review process to exclude another physician from practice, to restrict clinical privileges, or to otherwise harm the physician's practice.

Conflicts Between Members of a Health Care Team

All health professionals share a commitment to work together to serve the patient's interests. The best patient care is often a team effort, and mutual respect, cooperation, and communication should govern this effort. Each member of the patient care team has equal moral status. When a health professional has significant ethical objections to an attending physician's order, both should discuss the matter thoroughly. Mechanisms should be available in hospitals and outpatient settings to resolve differences of opinion among members of the patient care team. Ethics committees or ethics consultants may also be appropriate resources.

Research

Medical progress and improved patient care depend on innovative and vigorous research. Research is defined under the federal "Common Rule" as "a systematic investigation including research development, testing and evaluation, designed to develop or contribute to generalizable knowledge" (102). Honesty and integrity must govern all stages of research, from the initial design and grant application to publication of results. Investigators and their institutions are individually and jointly responsible for ensuring that the obligations of honesty and integrity are met. Fraud in research must be condemned and punished. Reviewers of grant applications and journal articles must respect the confidentiality of new ideas and information; they must not use what they learn from the review process for their own purposes, and they should not misrepresent the ideas of others as their own.

Scientists have a responsibility to gather data meticulously; to keep impeccable records; to interpret results objectively and not force them into preconceived molds or models; to submit their work to peer review; and to report new knowledge. Contributing to generalizable knowledge that can improve human health should be the main motivation for scientific research. Personal recognition, public acclaim, or financial gain should not be primary motivating factors, and physicians should be aware of conflicting interests when participating in or referring patients to research studies (103).

Human Subjects Research

The medical profession and individual researchers must assume responsibility for assuring that research is valid, has potentially significant value, and is ethically conducted. Research must be thoughtfully planned to ensure a high probability of useful results, to minimize subject risk and maximize subject safety, and to achieve a benefit-to-risk ratio high enough to justify the research effort (104). Benefits and risks of research must be distributed fairly, and particular care must be taken to avoid exploitation of vulnerable populations.

Functioning as both an investigator and the clinician of a patient-subject can result in conflict between what is best for the research protocol and what is in the patient's best interests. Physician-investigators should disclose this conflict to potential research participants and should maintain patient-subject health and welfare as their primary consideration (105). Patients should be informed that the primary motive of a research protocol is to gain new knowledge and that there may or may not be clinical benefit. It should also be clear to patients that participation in research is voluntary and not a requirement for continued clinical care.

Each research subject or an authorized representative (106) must be fully informed of the nature and risks of the research so that he or she may give truly informed consent to participate. Physicians have an ethical obligation to ensure that the informed consent information for a proposed research study is appropriate and understandable to the proposed subject population. Clinicians who are thinking about participating in or referring patients to research studies should be well versed about the responsible conduct of research and human subjects protections.

Independent review is a fundamental principle of ethical research. All proposed research, regardless of the source of support, must be assessed by an institutional review board to assure that the research plans are valid and reasonable, human subjects are adequately protected, the benefit-risk ratio is acceptable, the proposed research is sufficiently important and protective of human subjects in light of the local patient population, and the informed consent process and confidentiality protections are both appropriate and adequate. Physician-investigators and physicians referring patients to clinical studies have an independent professional obligation to satisfy themselves that those studies meet ethical standards.

While the formal independent review process was designed to protect research subjects, it cannot replace mutual trust and respect between subjects and researchers. Maintaining that trust and respect requires that physician-investigators involved in designing, performing, or referring patients to research studies have primary concern for the potential participants (107). If the risks of a study become too great or if continued participation cannot be justified, the physician must advise patients to withdraw. Physicians should not abdicate overall responsibility for patients they have referred to research studies.

Although the responsibility for assuring reasonable protection of human research subjects resides with the investigators and the institutional review board, the medical profession as a whole also has responsibilities. Clinical investigation is fraught with potential conflicts. Physicians should avoid situations in which they are rewarded for particular outcomes. Moreover, physicians who enroll their own patients in office-based research have an ethical obligation to disclose whether they have financial ties to sponsors (81,108). Giving or accepting finder's fees for referring patients to a research study generates an unethical conflict of interest for physicians (109). Compensation for the actual time, effort, and expense involved in research or recruiting patients is acceptable; any compensation above that level represents a profit and constitutes or can be perceived as an unethical conflict of interest.

While the Common Rule (110) and some state laws have provisions regarding privacy and confidentiality requirements for research, the HIPAA Privacy Rule now requires subject authorization for use or disclosure of protected health information for research. A Privacy Board can waive the authorization requirement or information can be used in a "limited data set" with a data use agreement or de-identified under HIPPA (111), although the HIPPA de-identification requirements are stricter than those under the Common Rule.

Physicians who engage in research studies or who make their patient records available for research purposes should be familiar with the HIPPA requirements and should protect their patients' trust by reviewing and approving each study's procedures for protecting data confidentiality and security.

Placebo Controls

Physicians may be asked to enroll patients in placebo-controlled trials. Although the World Medical Association requires that "the benefits, risks, burdens and effectiveness" of a new method be tested against the "best current prophylactic, diagnostic and therapeutic methods" (112), it deems placebo-controlled trials, despite the availability of proven therapy, to be only occasionally acceptable—namely, when compelling and scientifically sound methodological reasons require them or when the study involves a minor condition and patients receiving placebos will not be subject to additional risk for serious or irreversible harm (113).

This view, that control group members must receive standard, proven therapies, represents a change from the "gold standard" of the double-blind placebo-controlled trial. Another view is that physicians may ethically consider participating in or referring patients to placebo-controlled trials when participants freely consent to suspend knowledge of whether they are receiving effective treatment; the appropriateness of the study design has been reviewed and approved by an independent institutional review board (114) and: the health risks and consequences of placebo or delayed treatment are minimal; or the standard treatment offers no meaningful improvement to length or quality of life; or the available standard treatments are so toxic that patients routinely refuse therapy (115).

Before referring patients to a placebo-controlled study, a physician should ensure that the study design provides for monitoring his or her patients, unblinding treatment assignment to the referring physician, and withdrawing patients from the study if necessary.

Innovative Medical Therapies

The use of innovative medical therapies falls along the continuum between established practice and research. Innovative therapies include the use of unconventional dosages of standard medications, previously untried applications of known procedures, and the use of approved drugs for nonapproved indications. The primary purpose of innovative medical therapies is to benefit the individual patient. While medical innovations can yield important treatment results, they can also produce significant safety problems. Consequently, medical innovation should always be approached carefully. Medical therapy should be treated as research whenever data are gathered to develop new medical information and for publication. Adverse events should be carefully monitored. When considering an innovative therapy that has no precedent, the physician should consult with peers, an institutional review board, or other expert group to assess the risks, potential adverse outcomes, potential consequences of foregoing a standard therapy, and whether the innovation is in the patient's best interest (116). Informed consent is particularly important and requires that the patient understand that the recommended therapy is not standard treatment.

Scientific Publication and Public Announcements

Authors of research reports must be intimately acquainted with the work being reported so that they can take public responsibility for the integrity of the study and the validity of the findings. They must have substantially contributed to the research itself, and they must have been part of the decision to publish. Investigators must disclose project funding sources to potential research collaborators and publishers, and must explicitly inform publishers whether they do or do not have a potential conflict of interest (see the "Financial Conflicts of Interest" section). Physicians should not participate in privately funded research unless the sponsors confirm that they will not prevent the publication of negative results (117).

Scientists build on the published work of other researchers and can proceed with confidence only if they can rely on the accuracy of the previously reported results on which their work is based. All scientists have a professional responsibility to be honest when reporting their findings and when making public announcements of new research developments. Because media coverage of scientific developments can be fraught with misinterpretation, unjustified extrapolation and unwarranted conclusions, researchers should approach public pronouncements with extreme caution, using precise and measured language.

In general, press releases should be issued and press conferences held only after the research has been published in a peer-reviewed journal or presented in proper and complete abstract form so that the study details are available to the scientific community for evaluation. Statements of scientists receive great visibility. An announcement of preliminary results, even couched in the most careful terms, is frequently reported by the media as a "breakthrough." Spokespersons must avoid raising false public expectations or providing misleading information, both of which reduce the credibility of the scientific community as a whole.

Conclusion

The delivery of health care can pose challenging ethical dilemmas for patients, clinicians, and institutions. We hope that this Manual will help physicians, whether they are clinicians, educators, or researchers, to address these issues. The Manual is written for physicians by a physician organization as we attempt to navigate through difficult terrain. Our ultimate intent is to enhance the quality of care provided to patients. We hope the Manual will help thoughtful readers to be virtuous physicians, trusted by patients and the public.

Appendix: A Case Method To Assist with Clinical Ethics Decision Making

1. *Define the ethics problem as an "ought" or "should" question.*

Example: "Should we withhold a respirator for this unconscious adult man with AIDS, as his partner requests, or use it, as his parents request?"

Not: "This man with AIDS is an ethics problem."

Not: "Is it better for terminally ill patients to die with or without a respirator?"

2a. *List significant facts and uncertainties that are relevant to the question.* Include facts about the patient and caregivers (such as intimacy, emotional state, ethnic and cultural background, faith traditions, and legal standing).

Example: "This man and his partner have been living together for 10 years and purchased a house together. The partner has been a caregiver throughout the illness. The patient's parents have been unaccepting of his lifestyle and orientation and have been distant from him."

2b. *Include physiologic facts.*

Example: "The patient is irreversibly unconscious and incapable of making decisions; thus, he cannot now tell us who should speak on his behalf about his preferences for treatment."

2c. *Include significant medical uncertainties (such as prognosis and outcomes with and without treatment).*

Example: "Antibiotics can be given for the current lung infection, but we do not know whether the patient can be weaned from the respirator given the advanced disease. It seems more likely than not that he will eventually be weaned from the respirator. The patient has an estimated life span of 3 to 9 months, but it may be much shorter or somewhat longer."

2d. *Include the benefits and harms of the treatment options.*

Example: "The respirator will prolong life, but it is a burdensome and invasive treatment and will confine the patient to a highly medicalized setting."

3. *Identify a decision maker.* If the patient has decision-making capacity, the decision maker is the patient. If the patient lacks decision-making capacity,

identify a proxy decision maker as specified by court appointment, state law, a durable power of attorney for health care, living will, or the persons who are best situated by virtue of their intimate, loving familiarity with the patient.

Example: "This is a 32-year-old adult who has lived away from home for 14 years and who has had only occasional contact with his parents, mainly on holidays. He does not have a living will or a durable power of attorney but has spoken often with his partner about his preferences for health care as his disease has advanced. His partner has accompanied the patient to clinic and cared for him as he has become increasingly debilitated."

4. *Give understandable, relevant, desired information to the decision maker and dispel myths and misconceptions.*

Example: "The respirator and antibiotics will prolong life and may allow for treatment of the lung infection, but they will not reverse the underlying severity of the patient's condition. No existing treatments can affect this patient's underlying condition. If the respirator is started, it can be discontinued if the patient does not respond to treatment. If the respirator is not used, medications can be given to assure that the patient is comfortable even if his lungs are failing."

5. *Solicit values of the patient that are relevant to the question.* These include the patient's values about life; place in the life cycle; relation to community, health care, and health care institutions; goals for health care (for example, palliation, enhancement of function or independence, prolongation of life, or palliation without prolongation of life); and conditions that would change goals; and specific preferences about health care or proxy decision makers that are relevant to this situation.

Example: "This patient made many statements to his partner about wanting exclusively palliative care at this time and specifically declined further anti-HIV therapies, as noted in the medical record. He stated that he wanted no life-prolonging treatments of any kind if he could not communicate with his partner, which his present unconscious state prevents him from doing."

6. *Identify health professional values.* Values include health-promoting goals (such as prolonging life, alleviating pain, promoting health, curing disease, rehabilitating an injury, preventing harm, providing comfort, empowering patients to make choices, and advocating for patients). Values that pertain to patient-physician communication (truth telling, confidentiality, nondiscrimination, requirement for informed consent, and tolerance of the diversity of values) are also included, as well as some values that extend outside of the patient-physician relationship (such as protection of third parties, promotion of public health, and respect for the law).

Example: "Although the physician may feel that a respirator is indicated for this person with respiratory failure, this patient has articulated different goals for health care. The physician is obliged to respect the diversity of values and the requirement for informed consent and respect the patient's goals and preferences."

7. *Propose and critique solutions, including multiple options for treatment and alternative providers.*

Example: "The physician could provide palliative care to a person who has respiratory failure who elects not to receive a respirator or seek to expeditiously transfer the patient to someone who can provide such care (the latter course would disrupt a relationship between this physician and patient). The physician, in protecting the interests and values of this patient who cannot speak on his own behalf, must serve as the patient's advocate to the parents of the patient."

8. *Identify and remove or address constraints on solutions (such as reimbursement, unavailability of services, laws, or legal myths).*

Example: "The parents in this case asserted that the doctor had to obey them because they were family members. A check with the hospital attorney showed that this was not true in this state."

References

1. Peabody FW. The care of the patient. JAMA. 1927;88:877-82.

2. American College of Physicians Ethics Manual. Part 1: History; the patient; other physicians. American College of Physicians. Ann Intern Med. 1989;111:245-52. [PMID: 2665591]

3. American College of Physicians Ethics Manual. Part 2: The physician and society; research; life-sustaining treatment; other issues. American College of Physicians. Ann Intern Med. 1989;111:327-35. [PMID: 2757314]

4. Jonsen AR. The New Medicine and the Old Ethics. Cambridge, MA: Harvard Univ Pr; 1990.

5. Reiser SJ, Dyck AJ, Curran WJ. Ethics in Medicine: Historical Perspectives and Contemporary Concerns. Cambridge, MA: MIT Pr; 1977.

6. Rothman DJ. Strangers at the Bedside: A History of How Law and Bioethics Transformed Medical Decision Making. New York: Basic Books; 1991

7. Veatch RM. A Theory of Medical Ethics. New York: Basic Books; 1981.

8. Jonsen AR. The Birth of Bioethics. New York: Oxford Univ Pr; 1998.

9. Reich WT, ed. Encyclopedia of Bioethics. 2nd ed. New York: Macmillan; 1995.

10. Beauchamp TL, Childress JF. Principles of Biomedical Ethics. 5th ed. New York: Oxford Univ Pr; 2001.

11. President's Commission for the Study of Ethical Problems in Medicine and Biomedical and Behavioral Research. Making Health Care Decisions: A Report on the Ethical and Legal Implications of Informed Consent in the Patient-Practitioner Relationship. Washington, DC: President's Commission for the Study of Ethical Problems in Medicine and Biomedical and Behavioral Research; 1982.

12. Katz J. The Silent World of Doctor and Patient. New York: Free Pr; 1997.

13. President's Commission for the Study of Ethical Problems in Medicine and Biomedical and Behavioral Research. Securing Access to Health Care: A Report on the Ethical Implications of Differences in the Availability of Health Services. Washington, DC: President's Commission for the Study of Ethical Problems in Medicine and Biomedical and Behavioral Research; 1983.

14. President's Commission for the Study of Ethical Problems in Medicine and Biomedical and Behavioral Research. Screening and Counseling for Genetic Conditions: A Report on the Ethical, Social, and Legal Implications of Genetic Screening, Counseling, and Educational Programs. Washington, DC: President's Commission for the Study of Ethical Problems in Medicine and Biomedical and Behavioral Research; 1983.

15. President's Commission for the Study of Ethical Problems in Medicine and Biomedical and Behavioral Research. Splicing Life: A Report on the Social and Ethical Issues of Genetic Engineering with Human Beings. Washington, DC: President's Com-

mission for the Study of Ethical Problems in Medicine and Biomedical and Behavioral Research; 1982.

16. President's Commission for the Study of Ethical Problems in Medicine and Biomedical and Behavioral Research. Deciding to Forgo Life-Sustaining Treatment: A Report on the Ethical, Medical, and Legal Issues in Treatment Decisions. Washington, DC: President's Commission for the Study of Ethical Problems in Medicine and Biomedical and Behavioral Research; 1983.

17. Guidelines on the Termination of Life-Sustaining Treatment and the Care of the Dying. Briarcliff Manor, NY: The Hastings Center; 1987.

18. Medical professionalism in the new millennium: a physician charter. Ann Intern Med. 2002;136:243-6. [PMID: 11827500]

19. Snyder L, Tooker J. Obligations and opportunities: the role of clinical societies in the ethics of managed care. J Am Geriatr Soc. 1998;46:378-80. [PMID: 9514391]

20. American Medical Association. Guidelines for physician-patient electronic communications. Accessed at www.ama-assn.org/ama/pub/category/2386.html on 10 June 2004.

21. Snyder L, Weiner J. Ethics and Medicaid patients. In: Snyder L, ed. Ethical Choices: Case Studies for Medical Practice. 2nd ed. Philadelphia: American College of Physicians; 2005:130-5.

22. American Medical Association E-5.09. Confidentiality: Industry-Employed Physicians and Independent Medical Examiners.Chicago: American Medical Assoc; 1999.

23. American Medical Association E-10.03. Patient-Physician Relationship in the Context of Work-Related and Independent Medical Examinations. Chicago: American Medical Assoc; 1999.

24. U.S. Department of Health and Human Services. Privacy Rule, Standards for Privacy of Individually Identifiable Health Information. Code of Federal Regulations, Title 45, Part 46, Section 164: April 2001. To view the privacy rule and other information, see www.hhs.gov/ocr/hipaa.

25. Gostin LO. National health information privacy: regulations under the Health Insurance Portability and Accountability Act. JAMA. 2001;285:3015-21. [PMID: 11410101]

26. Health care needs of the adolescent. American College of Physicians. Ann Intern Med. 1989;110:930-5. [PMID: 2719425]

27. Burnum JF. Secrets about patients. N Engl J Med. 1991;324:1130-3. [PMID: 2008187]

28. Crawley LM, Marshall PA, Koenig BA. Respecting cultural differences at the end of life. In: Snyder L, Quill TE, eds. Physician's Guide to End-of-Life Care. Philadelphia: American College of Physicians–American Society of Internal Medicine; 2001:35-55.

29. Roter DL, Stewart M, Putnam SM, Lipkin M Jr, Stiles W, Inui TS. Communication patterns of primary care physicians. JAMA. 1997;277:350-6. [PMID: 9002500]

30. Quill TE, Townsend P. Bad news: delivery, dialogue, and dilemmas. Arch Intern Med. 1991;151:463-8. [PMID: 2001128]

31. Snyder L, Quill TE, eds. Physician's Guide to End of Care. Philadelphia: American College of Physicians; 2001.

32. Patient Education and Caring: End of Life (PEACE) Series. Philadelphia: Center for Ethics and Professionalism, American College of Physicians; 2001. Accessed at www.acponline.org/ethics/patient_education.htm.

33. Tobias BB, Ricer RE. Counseling adolescents about sexuality. Prim Care. 1998;25:49-70. [PMID: 9469916]

34. Geller G, Botkin JR, Green MJ, Press N, Biesecker BB, Wilfond B, et al. Genetic testing for susceptibility to adult-onset cancer. The process and content of informed consent. JAMA. 1997; 277:1467-74. [PMID: 9145720]

35. Rich EC, Burke W, Heaton CJ, Haga S, Pinsky L, Short MP, et al. Reconsidering the family history in primary care. J Gen Intern Med. 2004;19:273-80. [PMID: 15009784]

36. Weiner J. The duty to treat HIV-positive patients. In: Snyder L, ed. Ethical Choices: Case Studies for Medical Practice. 2nd ed. Philadelphia: American College of Physicians; 2005:136-42.

37. The acquired immunodeficiency syndrome (AIDS) and infection with the human immunodeficiency virus (HIV). Health and Public Policy Committee, American College of Physicians; and the Infectious Diseases Society of America. Ann Intern Med. 1988;108:460-9. [PMID: 3277519]

38. What is complementary and alternative medicine (CAM)? National Center for Complementary and Alternative Medicine, National Institutes of Health. Accessed at http://nccam.nih.gov/health/whatiscam#1 on 4 February 2005.

39. Berger JT. Multi-cultural considerations and the American College of Physicians Ethics Manual. J Clin Ethics. 2001;12:375-81. [PMID: 12026743]

40. Eisenberg DM, Davis RB, Ettner SL, Appel S, Wilkey S, Van Rompay M, et al. Trends in alternative medicine use in the United States, 1990-1997: results of a follow-up national survey. JAMA. 1998;280:1569-75. [PMID: 9820257]

41. The National Center for Complementary and Alternative Medicine, The National Institutes of Health. Accessed at www.nccam.nih.gov.

42. Carroll RJ. Should doctors treat their relatives? ACP–ASIM Observer. January 1999. Accessed at www.acponline.org/journals/news/jan99/relative.htm on 28 January 2005.

43. Eisenberg DM, Davis RB, Ettner SL, Appel S, Wilkey S, Van Rompay M, et al. Trends in alternative medicine use in the United States, 1990-1997: results of a follow-up national survey. JAMA. 1998;280:1569-75. [PMID: 9820257]

44. Weiner J, Tolle SW. Sex and the single physician. In: Snyder L, ed. Ethical Choices: Case Studies for Medical Practice. 2nd ed. Philadelphia: American College of Physicians; 2005:99-104.

45. Lyckholm LJ. Should physicians accept gifts from patients? JAMA. 1998;280:1944-6. [PMID: 9851481]

46. A controlled trial to improve care for seriously ill hospitalized patients. The study to understand prognoses and preferences for outcomes and risks of treatments (SUPPORT). The SUPPORT Principal Investigators. JAMA. 1995;274:1591-8. [PMID: 7474243]

47. Lo B, Quill T, Tulsky J. Discussing palliative care with patients. ACP-ASIM End-of-Life Care Consensus Panel. American College of Physicians-American Society of Internal Medicine. Ann Intern Med. 1999;130:744-9. [PMID: 10357694]

48. Institute of Medicine. Approaching Death: Improving Care at the End of Life. Washington, DC: National Academy Pr; 1997.

49. Cassel CK, Vladeck BC. ICD-9 code for palliative or terminal care. N Engl J Med. 1996;335:1232-4. [PMID: 8815949]

50. Buchan ML, Tolle SW. Pain relief for dying persons: dealing with physicians' fears and concerns. J Clin Ethics. 1995;6:53-61. [PMID: 7632997]

51. When you have pain at the end of life. Patient Education and Caring: End-of-Life (PEACE) Series. Philadelphia: American College of Physicians; 2001. Accessed at www.acponline.org/ethics/patient_education.htm on 28 January 2005.

52. Cassaret D, Kutner J, Abrahm J. Life after death: a practical approach to grief and bereavement. In: Snyder L, Quill TE, eds. Physician's Guide to End-of-Life Care. Philadelphia: American College of Physicians; 2001:178-93.

53. American College of Legal Medicine. Legal Medicine. 5th ed. St. Louis: Mosby; 2001.

54. Snyder L. Life, death, and the American College of Physicians: the Cruzan case [Editorial]. Ann Intern Med. 1990;112:802-4. [PMID: 2344110]

55. Annas GJ. The health care proxy and the living will. N Engl J Med. 1991;324:1210-3. [PMID: 2011167]

56. Physician Orders for Life-Sustaining Treatment (POLST). Accessed at www.ohsu.edu/ethics/polst/ on 28 January 2005.

57. Karlawish JH, Quill T, Meier DE. A consensus-based approach to providing palliative care to patients who lack decision-making capacity. ACP-ASIM End-of-Life Care Consensus Panel. American College of Physicians-American Society of Internal Medicine. Ann Intern Med. 1999;130:835-40. [PMID: 10366374]

58. Making medical decisions for a loved one at the end of life. Patient Education and Caring: End-of-Life (PEACE) Series. Philadelphia: American College of Physicians; 2001. Accessed at www.acponline.org/ethics/patient_education.htm on 28 January 2005.

59. Gazelle G. The slow code: should anyone rush to its defense? N Engl J Med. 1998;338:467-9. [PMID: 9459653]

60. Sabatino CP. Survey of state EMS-DNR laws and protocols. J Law Med Ethics. 1999;27:297-315, 294. [PMID: 11067612]

61. Herrin V, Poon P. Talking about organ procurement when one of your patients dies. ACP–ASIM Observer. February 2000. Accessed at www.acponline.org/ethics/casestudies/organ.htm on 28 January 2005.

62. Veatch RM. Transplantation Ethics. Washington, DC: Georgetown Univ Pr; 2000.

63. Williams MA, Lipsett PA, Rushton CH, Grochowski EC, Berkowitz ID, Mann SL, et al. The physician's role in discussing organ donation with families. Crit Care Med. 2003;31:1568-73. [PMID: 12771634]

64. Persistent vegetative state and the decision to withdraw or withhold life support. Council on Scientific Affairs and Council on Ethical and Judicial Affairs. JAMA. 1990;263:426-30. [PMID: 2403610]

65. Practice parameters: assessment and management of patients in the persistent vegetative state (summary statement). The Quality Standards Subcommittee of the American Academy of Neurology. Neurology. 1995;45:1015-8. [PMID: 7746375]

66. The vegetative state: guidance on diagnosis and management. Clin Med. 2003;3:249-54. [PMID: 12848260]

67. Withholding and withdrawing life-sustaining therapy. This Official Statement of the American Thoracic Society was adopted by the ATS Board of Directors, March 1991. Am Rev Respir Dis. 1991;144:726-31. [PMID: 1892317]

68. When Death Is Sought: Assisted Suicide and Euthanasia in the Medical Context. Albany, NY: New York State Task Force on Life and the Law; 1994.

69. Sulmasy DP, Pellegrino ED. The rule of double effect: clearing up the double talk. Arch Intern Med. 1999;159:545-50. [PMID: 10090110]

70. Quill TE, Byock IR. Responding to intractable terminal suffering: the role of terminal sedation and voluntary refusal of food and fluids. ACP-ASIM End-of-Life Care Consensus Panel. American College of Physicians-American Society of Internal Medicine. Ann Intern Med. 2000;132:408-14. [PMID: 10691593]

71. Snyder L, Sulmasy DP. Physician-assisted suicide. Ann Intern Med. 2001;135:209-16. [PMID: 11487490]

72. Hedberg K, Hopkins D, Kohn M. Five years of legal physician-assisted suicide in Oregon [Letter]. N Engl J Med. 2003;348: 961-4. [PMID: 12621146]

73. Sixth Annual Report on Oregon's Death with Dignity Act. 10 March 2004. Accessed at www.ohd.hr.state.or.us/chs/pas/ar-smmry.cfm on 28 January 2005.

74. Povar GJ, Blumen H, Daniel J, Daub S, Evans L, Holm RP, et al. Ethics in practice: managed care and the changing health care environment: medicine as a profession managed care ethics working group statement. Ann Intern Med. 2004;141:131-6. [PMID: 15262669]

75. Povar G, Moreno J. Hippocrates and the health maintenance organization. A discussion of ethical issues. Ann Intern Med. 1988;109:419-24. [PMID: 3136686]

76. LaPuma J, Schiedermayer D, Seigler M. Ethical issues in managed care. Trends Health Care Law Ethics. 1995;10:73-7. [PMID: 7655240]

77. Mechanic D, Schlesinger M. The impact of managed care on patients' trust in medical care and their physicians. JAMA. 1996;275:1693-7. [PMID: 8637148]

78. Braddock CH, Snyder L. Ethics and time, time perception and the patient-physician relationship. Position paper. Philadelphia: American College of Physicians; 2003.

79. Snyder L, Hillman AL. Financial incentives and physician decision making. In: Snyder L, ed. Ethical Choices: Case Studies for

Medical Practice. Philadelphia: American College of Physicians; 1996:105-12.

80. Sulmasy DP. Physicians, cost control, and ethics. Ann Intern Med. 1992;116:920-6. [PMID: 1580450]

81. Coyle SL. Physician-industry relations. Part 1: individual physicians. Ann Intern Med. 2002;136:396-402. [PMID: 11874314]

82. Conflicts of interest. Physician ownership of medical facilities. Council on Ethical and Judicial Affairs, American Medical Association. JAMA. 1992;267:2366-9. [PMID: 1564779]

83. Povar GJ, Snyder L. Selling products out of the office. Ethics and Human Rights Committee. Ann Intern Med. 1999;131:863-4. [PMID: 10610634]

84. Physicians and the pharmaceutical industry. American College of Physicians. Ann Intern Med. 1990;112:624-6. [PMID: 2327679]

85. The relationship between physicians and the pharmaceutical industry. A report of the Royal College of Physicians. J R Coll Physicians Lond. 1986;20:235-42. [PMID: 3534247]

86. Coyle SL, . Physician-industry relations. Part 2: organizational issues. Ann Intern Med. 2002;136:403-6. [PMID: 11874315]

87. Groman R, Ginsburg J. Racial and ethnic disparities in health care: a position paper of the American College of Physicians. Ann Intern Med. 2004;141:226-32. [PMID: 15289223]

88. Institute of Medicine. To Err Is Human: Building a Safer Health Care System. Washington, DC: National Academy Pr; 1999.

89. Tulsky JA, Snyder L. Deciding how much care is too much. ACP Observer. March 1997. Accessed at www.acponline.org/journals/news/mar97/howmuch.htm on 28 January 2005.

90. United Nations. First Congress on the Prevention of Crime and the Treatment of Offenders. Standard Minimum Rules for the Treatment of Prisoners. 1955. Accessed at www.unhchr.ch/html/menu3/b/h_comp34.htm on 28 January 2005.

91. National Commission on Correctional Health Care. Charging inmates a fee for health care services. 1996. Accessed at www.ncchc.org/resources/statements/healthfees.html on 28 January 2005.

92. Fletcher JC, Siegler M. What are the goals of ethics consultation? A consensus statement. J Clin Ethics. 1996;7:122-6. [PMID: 8889887]

93. Comprehensive Accreditation Manual for Hospitals: The Official Handbook. Oakbrook Terrace, IL: Joint Commission on Accreditation of Healthcare Organizations; 2004.

94. Aulisio MP, Arnold RM, Younger SJ. Health care ethics consultation: nature, goals, and competencies. A position paper from the Society for Health and Human Values-Society for Bioethics Consultation Task Force on Standards for Bioethics Consultation. Ann Intern Med. 2000;133:59-69. [PMID: 10877742]

95. Guidelines for the physician expert witness. American College of Physicians. Ann Intern Med. 1990;113:789. [PMID: 2240881]

96. Ginsburg J, Physicians and joint negotiations. Ann Intern Med. 2001;134:787-92. [PMID: 11329239]

97. Conley FK. Toward a more perfect world: eliminating sexual discrimination in academic medicine [Editorial]. N Engl J Med. 1993;328:351-2. [PMID: 8419824]

98. Crook ED, Weiner J. When residents and attendings disagree. In: Snyder L, ed. Ethical Choices: Case Studies for Medical Practice. 2nd ed. Philadelphia: American College of Physicians; 2005:148-53.

99. Snyder L. Referrals and patients wishes. In: Snyder L, ed. Ethical Choices: Case Studies for Medical Practice. 2nd ed. Philadelphia: American College of Physicians; 2005:77-81.

100. Weiner J, Snyder L. The impaired colleague. In: Snyder L, ed. Ethical Choices: Case Studies for Medical Practice. 2nd ed. Philadelphia: American College of Physicians; 2005:143-7.

101. Boisaubin EV, Levine RE. Identifying and assisting the impaired physician. Am J Med Sci. 2001;322:31-6. [PMID: 11465244]

102. Department of Health and Human Services. The Common Rule, Protection of Human Subjects. Code of Federal Regulations Title 45, Part 46.102 (d).

103. Commission on Research Integrity. Integrity and Misconduct in Research: Report to the Secretary of Health and Human Services, The House Committee on Commerce and the Senate Committee on Labor and Human Resources. Washington, DC: U.S. Department of Health and Human Services, Public Health Service; 1995.

104. Cassarett D, Snyder L, Karlawish J. When are industry-sponsored trials a good match for community doctors? ACP Observer. March 2001. Accessed at www.acponline.org/journals/news/mar01/ethics.htm on 28 January 2005.

105. Recruiting Human Subjects Sample Guidelines for Practice. Bethesda, MD: Department of Health and Human Services, Office of the Inspector General; June 2000. OEI-01-97-00196.

106. Cognitively impaired subjects. American College of Physicians. Ann Intern Med. 1989;111:843-8. [PMID: 2683918]

107. Drazen JM, Koski G. To protect those who serve [Editorial]. N Engl J Med. 2000;343:1643-5. [PMID: 11096176]

108. Bodenheimer T. Uneasy alliance: clinical investigators and the pharmaceutical industry. N Engl J Med. 2000;342:1539-44. [PMID: 10816196]

109. Lind SE. Finder's fees for research subjects. N Engl J Med. 1990;323:192-5. [PMID: 2362609]

110. Department of Health and Human Services. The Common Rule, Protection of Human Subjects. Code of Federal Regulations, Title 45, Part 46: Revised. 18 June 1991.

111. Protecting Personal Health Information in Research: Understanding the HIPAA Privacy Rule. Bethesda, MD: Department of Health and Human Services; 2003. NIH Publication no. 03-5388.

112. World Medical Association Declaration of Helsinki: ethical principles for medical research involving human subjects. JAMA. 2000;284:3043-5. [PMID: 11122593]

113. World Medical Association. Declaration of Helsinki. Ethical principles for medical research involving human subjects. For clarification to paragraph 29. 2002, see www.wma.net/e/policy/b3.htm.

114. Temple R, Ellenberg SS. Placebo-controlled trials and active-control trials in the evaluation of new treatments. Part 1: ethical and scientific issues. Ann Intern Med. 2000;133:455-63. [PMID: 10975964]

115. Amdur RJ, Bankert EA. The placebo-controlled clinical trial. In: Institutional Review Board Management and Function. Sudbury: Jones and Bartlett; 2002.

116. Lind SE. Innovative medical therapies: between practice and research. Clin Res. 1988;36:546-51. [PMID: 3180683]

117. International Committee of Medical Journal Editors. Uniform requirements for manuscripts submitted to biomedical journals. Updated October 2004. Accessed at www.icmje.org on 1 February 2005.

Index